Vegan Gluten-Free Cookbook

Easy To Make Vegan and Gluten-Free Recipes To Boost Your Mind And Body

Josephine M. Silva

WHAT IS IN THE BOOK?

INTRODUCTION 3
- WHAT IS THE VEGAN DIET? 6
- DIFFERENT TYPES OF VEGAN DIETS 9
- HEALTHY EATING AS A VEGAN 11
- FOODS TO EAT AND FOODS TO AVOID 18
- GOING GLUTEN-FREE 22
- BENEFITS OF GOING VEGAN AND GLUTEN-FREE 25

CHAPTER 1: BREAKFAST RECIPES 30
- SWISS CHARD CHICKPEA BREAKFAST SCRAMBLE 31
- VEGAN SCRAMBLED "EGGS" 34
- TOFU FRITTATA WITH SMOKY EGGPLANT SALSA 37
- EASY BREAKFAST PEACH COBBLER 41
- NUTRITION-RICH OMEGA 3 BLUEBERRY BREAKFAST COOKIES 44
- BUTTERNUT SQUASH BREAKFAST BOWL 48
- CHEESY QUINOA CUPS 51
- ALMOND AND PUMPKIN PORRIDGE 54

CHAPTER 2: LUNCH RECIPES 57
- ROOT VEGETABLE DAL 58
- VEGAN SKILLET ENCHILADAS 61
- CAULIFLOWER AND OYSTER MUSHROOM TACOS 65
- EGGPLANT CHICKPEA CURRY 69
- RED LENTIL CURRY SOUP 72
- MEDITERRANEAN LENTILS AND RICE 76
- QUINOA FALAFEL WITH AVOCADO TAHINI DRESSING 79
- ZUCCHINI NOODLES WITH PISTACHIO PESTO 82

CHAPTER 3: DINNER RECIPES 85
- FIG SPINACH SALAD WITH BALSAMIC VINAIGRETTE 86
- RICE, BEAN AND KALE BOWL WITH LEMON-DILL TAHINI 89

- CURRIED LENTILS WITH CARROTS AND CHICKPEAS 91
- MEXICAN TOFU SCRAMBLE 94
- THAI QUINOA SALAD WITH SESAME PEANUT SAUCE 97
- VEGGIE AND BEAN BURGERS 100
- CHICKPEA CRUST PIZZA 103
- ENCHILADAS VERDE 106

CHAPTER 4: SIDES AND SNACKS RECIPES 111

- CHICKPEA SALAD 112
- ZUCCHINI SQUARES 115
- LOW-CARB PIZZA STICKS 119
- SPICY BUFFALO CAULIFLOWER WINGS 122
- MISO SESAME KALE BOWL-ED OVER 125
- GREEN POWER BOWL 128
- RED LENTIL AND AMARANTH PROTEIN PATTIES 131
- BACON FLAVORED ROASTED CHICKPEAS 135

CHAPTER 5: DESSEERT RECIPES 138

- CHOCOLATE CHIP CHEWY BARS 139
- COFFEE CREAM BARS 142
- LEMON BLUEBERRY SWIRL CHEESECAKE SQUARES 145
- BLUEBERRY ICE CREAM 148
- HEALTHY HOLIDAY FUDGE 150
- PEANUT BUTTER OATMEAL ENERGY BITES 152
- PEANUT BUTTER CHOCOLATE CHIP COOKIES 155
- APPLE CRUMBLE MUFFINS 158

LAST WORDS 161

Copyright © 2018 by Josephine M. Silva- All rights reserved.

This document is geared towards providing exact and reliable information in regards to the topic and issue covered. The publication is sold with the idea that the publisher is not required to render accounting, officially permitted, or otherwise, qualified services. If advice is necessary, legal or professional, a practiced individual in the profession should be ordered.

From a Declaration of Principles which was accepted and approved equally by a Committee of the American Bar Association and a Committee of Publishers and Associations.

In no way is it legal to reproduce, duplicate, or transmit any part of this document by either electronic means or in printed format. Recording of this publication is strictly prohibited, and any storage of this document is not allowed unless with written permission from the publisher. All rights reserved.

The information provided herein is stated to be truthful and consistent, in that any liability, in terms of inattention or otherwise, by any usage or abuse of any policies, processes, or directions contained within is the solitary and utter responsibility of the recipient reader. Under no circumstances will any legal responsibility or blame be held against the publisher for any reparation, damages, or monetary loss due to the information herein, either directly or indirectly.

Respective authors own all copyrights not held by the publisher.

The information herein is offered for informational purposes solely and is universal as so. The presentation of the information is without contract or any type of guarantee assurance.

The trademarks that are used are without any consent, and the publication of the trademark is without permission or backing by the trademark owner. All trademarks and brands within this book are for clarifying purposes only and are owned by the owners themselves, not affiliated with this document.

INTRODUCTION

Increasingly more people have decided to go vegan for environmental, ethical and health reasons. Since you are reading this book, you might very well be considering how to go vegan and understand the changes you will need to make in your diet and lifestyle. First, you should understand that the vegan diet can help you turn your body around, reach your ideal weight and boost both your body and mind as it has already for millions of people before you.

When done right, a vegan dieting plan can result in numerous positive health benefits including improved blood sugar control and a trimmer waistline. This book will guide you through the most important steps you have to take to convert to a vegan diet. You will also learn delicious vegan, gluten-free recipes that will additionally boost your weight loss as you move towards your ideal weight.

Included in this book, you will also find important information you must know before you switch to vegan. Therefore, it will act as a guide to help you on this weight loss and life changing conversion. So, let's begin.

WHAT IS THE VEGAN DIET?

Veganism is commonly defined as a way of living which attempts to completely exclude all forms of animal cruelty and exploitation whether for food or other purposes. For these reasons, going vegan means you must eliminate all animal products from your diet including dairy, eggs, and meat. People decide to go vegan for many reasons commonly ranging from environmental to ethical concerns.

Whatever the reason, people also find that veganism improves their overall state of health.

Where veganism was once something strange and reserved for groups like those peace-loving hippies of long ago, it has since come a long way. More and more people every day show interests in following a totally animal-free diet with many celebrities leading the charge.

However, before you decide to jump on the no-meat-eggs-and-dairy bandwagon, you should know what you are getting into. Keep in mind that adopting a vegan lifestyle comes with obstacles and requires constant planning. You must plan and track nutrients like proteins to ensure you are getting the amounts your body needs.

Unlike a vegetarian approach that only excludes meat, a vegan approach eliminates all animal foods including dairy and eggs. Therefore, all vegan meals are based on grains, vegetables, fruit, nuts, seeds and other dairy alternatives like soy, which is high in fiber and low in protein.

Therefore, a vegan diet includes only plants like grains, nuts and fruits and other foods made from plants. However, do not worry, with good planning as well as understanding of what makes up a balanced and healthy vegan diet, you will get all required nutrients.

Especially, once you prepare delicious meals from the book. By following a varied as well as balanced vegan diet, you will be able to get the required nutrients you need from your foods. It may be difficult at the very beginning, but once your body gets used to the new dieting approach, you will start enjoying the new you.

DIFFERENT TYPES OF VEGAN DIETS

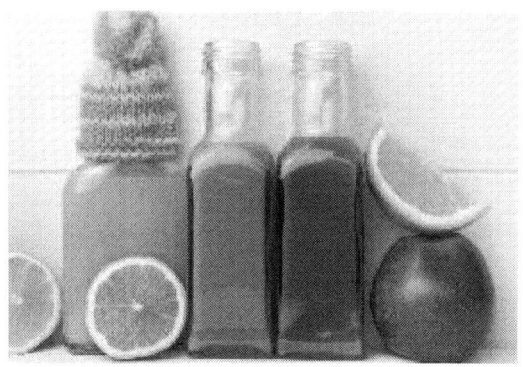

There are several types of vegan diets. The most common include raw-food vegan diet, whole-food vegan diet, 80/10/10, the starch solution vegan diet, junk-food vegan diet and raw till 4.

Whole-food vegan diet is a diet based on a wide range of whole plant foods including whole grains, seeds, nuts, fruits, and vegetables while raw-food vegan diet is based on raw vegetables, fruits, seeds, nuts and plant food, which are cooked at temperatures below 118°F.

Another common type of vegan dieting plan is 80/10/10 that is a raw-food vegan diet which mainly limits those fat-rich plants like avocados and nuts to rely commonly on those soft greens and raw fruits instead. Therefore, this vegan diet is also commonly referred to as the raw-food, low-fat vegan diet or fruitarian diet.

There is also the starch solution vegan diet that includes high-carb and low-fat foods mainly focused on those cooked starches like rice, corn, and potatoes instead of fruits. Raw till 4 is another common type of vegan diet which is primarily inspired by the starch solution and 80/10/10. Following this vegan diet means you must consume raw foods until 4 p.m. You also have an option to consume cooked plant-based meals after 4 p.m. for dinner.

The last type of vegan diet is the junk-food vegan diet that is lacking in whole plant foods. It mainly relies on cheeses, mock meats, vegan desserts, fries and other heavily processed vegan meals.

Even though there are several vegan dieting plans, most scientific research rarely differentiates between these types. Therefore, the information and details in the book relate to all the different types of vegan dieting plans, as there are little or no differences between them.

HEALTHY EATING AS A VEGAN

You will be able to get most of the nutrients your body needs by eating a balanced and varied vegan diet. To follow a healthy vegan diet, make sure you eat at least five portions of vegetables and fruit every day. In addition, base your meals on bread, pasta, rice, potatoes and other starchy carbohydrates. Choose whole grain whenever possible.

You also need to provide dairy alternatives like yogurts and soy drinks, just make sure you choose lower-sugar and lower-fat options.

In addition, eat some pulses, beans and other protein-rich foods. Pulses are the dried edible seeds of certain plants in the legume family. You also should include unsaturated spreads and oils and eat them in smaller portions every day. Keep in mind to drink plenty of fluids as well since the recommended amount is six to eight cups or glasses per day.

If you are consuming drinks and foods which are high in sugar, salt or fat, make sure you have these less often and in smaller portions. Therefore, with good planning, you can get all the required nutrients your body needs from vegan meals.

In addition, keep in mind to eat foods rich in vitamin D and calcium like unsweetened soya, oat and rice drinks. You may also consume calcium-set tofu, tahini and sesame seeds, plenty of pulses, white and brown bread, and dried fruits like figs, dried apricots, raisins and prunes.

To get enough iron, you should eat pulses, whole meal flour or bread, breakfast cereals loaded with iron, some dark-green leafy vegetables like broccoli, spring greens and watercress, nuts and dried fruits.

When it comes to the source of vitamin B12, make sure you eat plenty of breakfast cereals loaded with B12, unsweetened soya drinks, yeast extracts like Marmite, which is loaded with vitamin B12. Then, you must focus on consuming foods that include omega-3 fatty acids like linseed or flaxseed oil, grapeseed oil, walnuts, soya oil and soy-based food like tofu.

Therefore, you will need a B12 supplement as vitamin B12 naturally occurs only in animal foods.

Therefore, stock up on a variety of these vitamin B12-fortified foods and some other vitamin B12 supplements.

Keep in mind that vitamin B12 keeps the body's blood and nerve cells healthy helping making DNA, so deficiencies in this vitamin can lead to weakness, tiredness, loss of appetite, weight loss, constipation, various nerve problems, anxiety and depression.

As already mentioned, you must consume foods rich in iron. At some point, you may need an iron supplement as well. Iron comes in two forms, non-Heme and Heme. Heme makes up about forty percent of the iron in animal foods that the body easily absorbs.

However, vegan diets contain only those non-Heme irons that are less readily absorbed, meaning you must ingest more iron for the body to gain the benefits from it. Some good iron sources include sunflower seeds, dark leafy greens, legumes and dried raisins.

Then, once you start following a vegan diet, you will have to find new protein sources. Proteins are the main building blocks of life, so every diet should contain protein as said by every vegan dietitian. Proteins in our bodies break down into amino acids, which promote cell repair and cell growth.

You should consume at least 0.8 grams of protein daily for every kilogram of body mass, which is around 54 grams of proteins for a 150-pound woman. The best vegan sources of protein include lentils, beans, natural soy, quinoa and seitan.

In addition, keep in mind that you should not entirely replace animal products with junk. Swapping out meat for pasta, white bread and other packaged foods set you up for a major failure. It is not a good idea to trade those animal products for processed foods which provide little nutritional value. The main results of this approach are a grumpier mood, hunger and weight gain.

In addition, remember to take it easy on those soy-based products. Once you start following a vegan diet, you must carefully plan your meals and include a wide range of different foods that are allowable on a vegan diet.

Therefore, consuming too much of those soy-based vegan meals is worse than consuming those high-quality animal products. In addition, meat substitutes are often loaded with preservatives and highly-processed, so always read labels carefully.

The healthiest sources of soy include tofu, miso, tempeh, edamame and soy milk.

Moreover, bear in mind that you do not have to make this switch all at once. It really takes work, planning and really understanding what a balanced and varied vegan diet looks like. It also takes time for your body to get used to this newly initiated diet plan. Therefore, make gradual changes before you focus on a vegan dieting entirely.

FOODS TO EAT AND FOODS TO AVOID

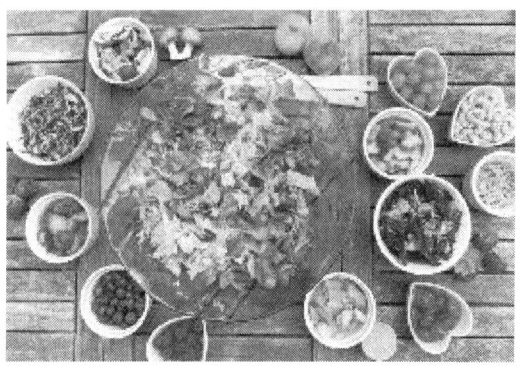

Foods to eat while following a vegan diet include those vegan animal product substitutes with plant-based replacements including tempeh, tofu, and seitan that provide versatile protein-rich alternatives to meals like eggs, fish, and poultry in many recipes.

You should also consume legumes like beans, peas, and lentils, which are excellent sources of nutrients and beneficial plant compounds. In addition, keep in mind that fermenting, sprouting and proper cooking can greatly increase nutrient absorption.

You should eat nuts and nut butters especially those made of unroasted and unbleached varieties that are great sources of fiber, iron, magnesium, selenium, vitamin E, and zinc.

When it comes to seeds, consume chia, flaxseed, and hemp that contain a liberal amount of beneficial omega-3 fatty acids and proteins. You should also consume calcium-fortified yogurts and plant links as these can help you achieve the recommended dietary daily calcium intake. Make sure you opt for selections that are fortified with vitamin D and vitamin B12 whenever possible.

Other amazing sources of complete protein are algae including chlorella and spirulina. Other algae varieties are also great iodine sources you should include in your dieting plan.

Once you go vegan, make sure you consume nutritional yeast, which is the easiest way of increasing the protein content of your vegan meals and add that tasty and interesting cheesy flavor. In addition, pick those vitamin B12-fortified varieties whenever you can.

Cereals, whole grains, and pseudo-cereals are also more than welcome when you follow a vegan diet as these are great sources of fiber, complex carbs, iron, minerals and B vitamins.

Other high-protein options include teff, quinoa, spelt and amaranth. You can also consume fermented and sprouted plant foods including miso, pickles, natto, tempeh, Ezekiel, kimchi and kombucha, which often contain vitamin K2 and probiotics. Keep in mind that fermenting and sprouting these foods can improve their mineral absorption.

In addition, eat plenty of vegetables and fruit as both are great for your body when it comes to increasing the daily nutrient intake. Therefore, consume a lot of spinach, kale, bok choy, watercress and other leafy greens especially those high in calcium and iron. Remember that these minimally processed plant foods are the best additions to any vegan refrigerator.

When it comes to those foods you should avoid, you should not eat poultry and meat including organ meats, chicken, goose, duck, pork, veal, beef and other. You must avoid seafood and fish including all types of fish like squid, scallops, crab, mussels, calamari, anchovies, lobster and other.

You also must avoid consuming dairy products like butter, ice cream, yogurt, milk, and cheese. Eggs from ostriches, fish, chickens, and quails are also forbidden as well as bee products like bee pollen, honey and royal jelly.

You must also avoid those animal-based ingredients like lactose, whey, casein, egg white albumen, cochineal or carmine, shellac, animal-derived vitamin D3, gelatin, isinglass, L-cysteine and those fish-derived omega 3-fatty acids. The bottom line is you should avoid consuming any animal by-products, animal flesh, and foods that contain ingredients from animal origin.

GOING GLUTEN-FREE

Gluten is a general name for those proteins found in wheat products like rye, barley, spelt, faro and other wheat derivatives. Gluten mainly helps food maintain its shape. In fact, it acts as glue, which holds foods together. It can be found in various types of foods like bread, pasta, sauces, roux, salad dressings, baked goods, soups, cereals and others.

Fortunately, there are many delicious foods you can eat which are naturally gluten-free. There are also many grain foods which are naturally gluten-free that you can enjoy in a wide range of interesting and creative ways.

At first, cutting gluten from your diet may seem like a difficult task. However, there are many healthy, delicious foods you can consume that are naturally gluten-free. The most healthy and cost-effective way to follow a vegan, gluten-free diet is to consume those foods, which are naturally gluten-free like vegetables, fruits, beans, legumes, and nuts.

Things like pure wheat grass and barley grass that can be found naturally gluten-free are good to consume. Other starch-containing foods which are naturally gluten-free like rice, beans, quinoa, amaranth, chia, arrowroot, tapioca, potato, soy, cassava, corn, beans, teff, flax, gluten-free oats and nut flours are also good to eat on this diet. You also may consume gluten-free substitutes like gluten-free bread and other products free of gluten. Combined with a vegan diet, you should base your diet mainly on vegetables, fruits and other healthy foods groups listed above.

It is common that the traditional wheat foods like bread, crackers, pasta and various baked goods are usually not gluten-free. However, you can find many gluten-free options of these foods you can use as alternative grains and flours. There are also gluten-free flours, so you can make your own bread that is gluten-free. You can also eat gluten-free cereals and oats. These foods typically contain gluten, but there are numerous varieties of these foods you can purchase that are gluten-free.

Also, both fresh and frozen vegetables and fruits are naturally gluten-free, so make sure you include plenty of these foods in your diet. In addition, most beverages are also gluten-free like juices, sports drinks, and sodas. On the other hand, beverages like lagers, beers, ales and malt vinegar are not gluten-free, so make sure you avoid them.

BENEFITS OF GOING VEGAN AND GLUTEN-FREE

There are numerous benefits of going vegan and gluten-free. You can enjoy these benefits as soon as you embark on this adventurous, healthier, lifestyle journey. Vegan diet, for instance, can help you lose weight and lower your body mass index in a couple of weeks after beginning.

Since vegan diets can help people lose weight, it is no wonder why more and more people decide to go vegan each day. Other weight-related benefits of vegan diets include healthier lifestyle choices like energy for more physical activity and other health-related behaviors.

There have been numerous studies conducted about veganism that indicate following a vegan diet is a much more effective way to lose weight than other similar dieting alternatives.

Therefore, vegan diets are more effective when it comes to helping people naturally reduce their daily calorie intake. This fact eventually results in weight loss meaning that people following vegan diets are much more satisfied with their bodies and weight.

Going vegan and gluten-free can also help you keep your blood sugar in check and avoid Type 2 Diabetes.

There are studies that have shown that most vegans benefit from significantly lower blood sugar levels, higher insulin sensitivity, and a seventy-eight percent lower risk of developing serious health conditions like Type 2 Diabetes than those people who are non-vegans. This statistic included pre-diabetics and existing diabetics making their lives easier as they worked to avoid their diabetes symptoms.

A portion of these advantages can be explained by the higher fiber intake that may result in the positive blood sugar response. Therefore, vegan diets both lower your blood sugar levels and lead you towards weight loss, so eventually, you can enjoy watching your body transform.

A vegan diet and gluten-free diet combined can also help you keep your heart healthy. Studies have shown that vegans may have up to seventy-five lower risk of developing high blood pressure and around forty-two percent lower risk of developing heart disease. Therefore, vegan diets are very effective at both reducing cholesterol and blood sugar levels leading you towards a better state of mind and body. These effects are especially beneficial as by reducing your blood sugar levels and cholesterol levels, you are also lowering the risk of developing heart disease.

Other benefits of going vegan and gluten-free include a fifteen percent lower risk of developing cancer, reducing symptoms of arthritis like joint swelling, morning stiffness, and pain, reducing the risk of poor kidney functions and reducing the risk of developing Alzheimer's disease.

Knowing these facts, you should make the decision to proceed on this adventurous journey right away. Going vegan and gluten-free does not have to be challenging especially once you try the delicious recipes listed here in this book.

No matter what your reasons for deciding to turn to veganism and gluten-free diets, you will enjoy being more energized. You will also enjoy seeing the improvements to your body weight and the benefits to your health.

CHAPTER 1: BREAKFAST RECIPES

Going vegan and gluten-free at the very beginning may seem like a very difficult task as you must completely change your lifestyle and your dieting. However, there are plenty of delicious foods you can enjoy every day without hunger and deprivation. It may be hard at first to get used to eating vegan meals, but once your body becomes accustomed to your new dieting plan, you will feel better than ever.

Keep in mind that going vegan also helps you lose weight, so after several weeks of following a vegan diet expect to lose additional pounds and move closer toward your ideal body weight.

SWISS CHARD CHICKPEA BREAKFAST SCRAMBLE

If you are looking for an easy to prepare, delicious vegan and gluten-free meal, I suggest you make this amazingly delicious Swiss chard chickpea breakfast scramble loaded with nutrients to properly start your day.

Nutritional information for one serving:

- Total Calories: 212
- Protein: 7 grams
- Fat: 4 grams
- Fiber: 6 grams
- Carbohydrates: 32 grams

Ingredients:

- 1 tablespoon of coconut oil
- 1/2 white onion, sliced thinly
- 4-5 cloves of minced garlic
- 1 can of chickpeas, drained and rinsed
- 2 tablespoons of nutritional yeast
- Juice from half lemon
- 1 teaspoon of turmeric
- 3 large leaves of Swiss Chard with stems removed, roughly chopped
- Optional for topping avocado, hemp hearts, flax seeds and nutritional yeast

Method:

1. The initial step is to heat oil in a skillet placed over medium heat. Once the oil is melted, add garlic and onions and sauté for about five minutes until onions are entirely fragrant and translucent.

2. In the meantime, while the onions are cooking, place chickpeas in a small bowl along with the fresh lemon juice, nutritional yeast, salt and turmeric.

3. Then stir ingredients together well as you partially mash chickpeas. However, make sure you leave most of them whole.

4. Once done, transfer seasoned chickpeas to the skillet and cook for at least three minutes. Then, stir in Swiss Chard until slightly wilted and soft.

5. Serve the meal immediately with preferred toppings and enjoy.

VEGAN SCRAMBLED "EGGS"

If you have been a vegan for quite some time, you probably miss those delicious scrambled eggs you used to eat every morning. Well, you do not have to miss them, because you can prepare astonishingly delightful vegan scrambled eggs which are the perfect vegan option for eggs.

Nutritional information for one serving:

- Total Calories: 278
- Protein: 18.5 grams
- Fat: 20.5 grams
- Fiber: 0.2 grams
- Carbohydrates: 9 grams

Ingredients:

- 1 tablespoon of coconut oil
- 1/4 cup of diced white onion

- 2 cloves of minced garlic
- 6 oz. of extra firm tofu
- 1/4 cup of nutritional yeast
- Juice of half lemon
- Salt and pepper to taste

Method:

1. The initial step is to heat the coconut oil using a small skillet placed over medium to high heat.

2. Once done, add garlic and diced onion and sauté until fragrant and gold. This will take about five minutes.

3. In the meantime, while the onions and garlic are sautéing, crumble tofu in a small bowl using your fingers.

4. Once done, stir in lemon juice, nutritional yeast, salt and pepper.

5. The following step is to add tofu mixture to the onion mixture and cook for about three minutes until tofu is entirely heated.

6. Once done, serve the meal and enjoy.

TOFU FRITTATA WITH SMOKY EGGPLANT SALSA

This vegan, gluten-free breakfast dish is easy to put together and preparing it in the morning will not take much time when you are running around trying to get ready to go to work.

Nutritional information for one serving:

- Total Calories: 190
- Protein: 8 grams
- Fat: 5 grams
- Fiber: 7 grams
- Carbohydrates: 31 grams

Ingredients:

- 1 package of Extra Firm Tofu, water packed
- 1/3 cup of unsweetened nondairy milk
- 1 tablespoon of cornstarch

- 3 tablespoons of nutritional yeast
- 1 teaspoon of ground mustard
- 2 teaspoons of turmeric
- 1 diced red pepper
- 1 fine diced small onion
- 2 small potatoes, diced
- 1 tablespoon of olive oil
- 2 cloves of garlic
- Salt and pepper
- For eggplant salsa: 1 medium eggplant
- 2 cloves of garlic
- 1 tablespoon of extra virgin olive oil
- 2 small tomatoes, diced
- 1/2 teaspoon of smoked paprika
- 1/4 cup of red wine vinegar
- 1/3 cup of diced cilantro
- Salt and pepper

Method:

1. The initial step is to preheat the oven to 375 degrees and prepare a pie dish by spraying it with non-stick cooking spray. Use parchment paper and cut a circle the same size as the dish and place it inside. Set dish aside.

2. The following step is to heat a small skillet placed over medium to high heat. Then, add garlic and oil. About two minutes later, add in the pepper, potatoes and onions. Sauté about ten minutes until vegetables are soft and tender.

3. The next step is to put the tofu dry and crumbled using a food processor. Once tofu is crumbled, add in the turmeric, nutritional yeast, cornstarch, almond milk, salt, mustard and pepper. Process until all ingredients are smooth and well combined.

4. Then, prepare a large bowl, pour in the tofu mixture and add vegetables. Mix well and pour into the already prepared pie dish.
5. Bake for about forty minutes until the top of the frittata is firm to the touch. Once baking has completed, let it cool.

6. Prepare a medium skillet and heat oil placed over medium to high heat. Then, add in eggplant and sauté for about five minutes until eggplant has a slight crisp on the outside. Then pour eggplant into a bowl and add in the remaining eggplant salsa ingredients.

7. Season the meal with salt and pepper, serve and enjoy.

EASY BREAKFAST PEACH COBBLER

This wonderfully scrumptious vegan, gluten-free meal is like having the best dessert for breakfast every morning. It is so tasty and has only 195 calories per serving, so your weight loss progress will not be spoiled.

Nutritional information for one serving:

- Total Calories: 195
- Protein: 3 grams
- Fat: 7 grams
- Fiber: 6 grams
- Carbohydrates: 31 grams

Ingredients:

- 2 cups plus 2 tablespoons of gluten-free oats
- 1/2 teaspoon of sea salt
- 3 tablespoons of coconut oil, solid

- 1/4 cup of agave nectar or maple syrup
- 1/2 cup of unsweetened almond milk
- For peach filling 15 oz. cans of Libby's Yellow Cling Peach Sliced, drained thoroughly
- 2 teaspoons of ground cinnamon
- 1/2 teaspoon of ground nutmeg
- 1/4 teaspoon of sea salt
- 2 tablespoons of lemon juice
- 2 tablespoons of oat flour
- 2 tablespoons of maple syrup, optional

Method:

1. The initial step is to preheat the oven to 350 degrees. Then, grease a cast-iron skillet very lightly with coconut oil. Set the skillet aside.

2. The following step is to use a food processor to blend the oats until it reaches a flour-like consistency. Set aside.

3. The next step is to prepare a 10-inch cast iron skillet and add in all the ingredients

listed for the peach filling alongside two tablespoons of oat flour. Once done, stir well to combine all ingredients.

4. Then, in the food processor, add the sea salt and blend again. Then, add in the coconut milk and cut it into the flour consistency. Once complete, add in maple syrup or agave nectar and almond milk. Pulse until a wet dough comes together.

5. Then, spoon the dough mixture over the peach filling. Bake for at least thirty to thirty-five minutes until the cobbler topping is all set.

6. Remove from the oven and cool slightly. Once cooled, serve it with an extra drizzle of maple syrup and coconut creams. You may add more fruits as well.

NUTRITION-RICH OMEGA 3 BLUEBERRY BREAKFAST COOKIES

This is a fantastic breakfast recipe you can prepare easily and quickly. You will love the idea of having tasty cookies for breakfast. Make sure you make a bunch of them, as your family members will ask for more.

Nutritional information for one serving:

- Total Calories: 206
- Protein: 4.9 grams
- Fat: 12.2 grams
- Fiber: 4.5 grams
- Carbohydrates: 22.8 grams

Ingredients:

- 2 tablespoons of melted coconut oil
- 1/4 cup of coconut sugar
- 1 medium banana, mashed
- 1/2 teaspoon of vanilla extract
- 1/2 teaspoon of almond extract
- 1/4 cup of flaxseed meal
- 1/2 cup of almond meal or flour
- 1/2 teaspoon of baking soda
- 1/2 teaspoon of cinnamon
- 1/4 teaspoon of salt
- 1 1/4 cups of rolled gluten-free oats
- 1 tablespoon of chia seeds
- 1/2 cup of fresh or frozen blueberries
- 1/4 cup of chopped walnuts
- 2 oz.- of chopped vegan dark chocolate, optional

Method:

1. The initial step is to preheat the oven to 350 degrees. Then, line a large baking sheet with parchment paper to prevent sticking.

2. The following step is to mix together coconut sugar, melted coconut oil, almond extracts vanilla and mashed banana in a large bowl until creamy and smooth.

3. The next step is to fold in almond meal, flaxseed meal, salt, baking soda and cinnamon and mix until a thick dough forms.

4. Next, add in chia seeds and oats and gently fold into the butter until all ingredients are evenly distributed.

5. Lastly, fold in walnuts, blueberries and dark chocolate if using.

6. Use a large cookie dough spoon to scoop dough onto already prepared cookie sheet. Make sure to gently press them onto the sheet.

7. Bake for at least fifteen minutes until edges become golden brown.

8. Make sure to allow the cookies to slightly cool down before you remove them from the pan and serve. The ingredients listed make ten big cookies.

BUTTERNUT SQUASH BREAKFAST BOWL

If you love to enjoy light meals in the morning that are easy to prepare and literally done in minutes, consider preparing this surprisingly delectable vegan, gluten-free butternut squash breakfast bowl loaded with nutrients.

Nutritional information for one serving:

- Total Calories: 157
- Protein: 3 grams
- Fat: 11 grams
- Fiber: 6 grams
- Carbohydrates: 15 grams

Ingredients:

- 1 tablespoon of coconut oil
- 12 oz. of butternut squash, cubed, frozen or fresh
- 1 tablespoon of peanut butter
- 1/4 teaspoon of cinnamon
- 1/4 teaspoon of all-spice
- 2 teaspoon of maple syrup

Method:

1. The initial step is to warm the oil placed over medium heat. Once done, add in the butternut squash.

2. Cook until it begins to soften if using fresh, or until it is warm through if using frozen. Either way, this will take around eight minutes.

3. The next step is to add in the remaining ingredients and stir everything well. Let it cook for at least three minutes. Then, serve the meal warm and enjoy.

CHEESY QUINOA CUPS

This remarkably appetizing recipe keeps the essence of eggy breakfast cups, but the eggs are replaced with tasty chickpea flour loaded with delicious cheese for nutritional yeast. This meal is loaded with nutrients the body needs to jump start your day properly.

Nutritional information for one serving:

- Total Calories: 189
- Protein:52 grams
- Fat: 10 grams
- Fiber: 7 grams
- Carbohydrates: 19 grams

Ingredients:

- 1 cup of non-dairy milk
- 1/3 cup of chickpea flour
- 2 tablespoons of nutritional yeast
- 2 tablespoons of olive oil
- 1/4 teaspoon of fine sea salt
- 1/8 teaspoon of turmeric, optional
- 1 1/2 cups of cooked quinoa
- 1/2 cup of chopped green onions
- 1 cup of vegan cheddar cheese

Method:

1. Start with preparing a large bowl. Whisk the chickpea flour, salt, olive oil, yeast, turmeric if using, until smooth. Then, loosely cover the bowl and let it stand for at least thirty minutes. You may refrigerate it up to twenty-four hours.

2. The following step is to preheat the oven to 375 degrees. Then, grease or line six cups of a standard muffin tin.

3. The next step is to add the quinoa and two tablespoons of the green onions to the chickpea batter. Then, divide the mixture evenly between the already prepared muffin cups. Divide cheese evenly among the cups as well. Make sure to press it gently into batter. Once done, sprinkle the cups with remaining green onions.

4. Bake in the preheated oven for at least twenty minutes until the centers are set. Then transfer the muffin tin to a cooling rack and let it cool for about fifteen minutes.

5. Remove the muffins from the tin. Serve warm and enjoy.

ALMOND AND PUMPKIN PORRIDGE

You are going to absolutely love this breakfast porridge made of almond and sweet potatoes. This is an incredibly mouthwatering and simple meal to make. It is perfect for those busy mornings when you do not have a lot of time to spend fixing breakfast.

Nutritional information for one serving:

- Total Calories: 250
- Protein: 7 grams
- Fat: 11 grams
- Fiber: 6 grams
- Carbohydrates: 35 grams

Ingredients:

- 1 cup of canned pumpkin, you may use homemade pumpkin puree as well
- 1/3 cup of almond pulp, leftover from homemade almond milk
- 1 heaping tablespoon of chia seed or ground flax
- 1/3 cup of almond milk
- Pinch of sea salt
- 1/2 teaspoon of ground cinnamon
- 2 tablespoons of maple syrup, if desired
- For topping: chopped nuts, cacao, dried fruit and nibs

Method:

1. The initial step is to add the pulp, pumpkin, chia or flax meal, almond milk, cinnamon and sea salt to a small saucepan.

2. The next step is to whisk all ingredients well mixed. Then place the pan over medium heat until ingredients start to bubble.

3. Reduce heat to low and let the porridge simmer gently for several minutes as you stir frequently.

4. Remove the pot from the heat and drizzle with maple syrup, if using. Sprinkle on the toppings you prefer. Serve and enjoy. The ingredients listed are for a single serving.

CHAPTER 2: LUNCH RECIPES

In the following section of the book, you are going to learn some amazing vegan, gluten-free lunch recipes. You will absolutely love them especially as they are very simple to make and do not take a lot of prep time. Thanks to these recipes and the delicious meals you can eat, vegan and gluten-free diets do not have to difficult and challenging as you lose weight as you go.

Once your body has adapted and learns to accept your new healthy lifestyle, you will see a recognizable weight loss, and experience feeling healthier in just several weeks of starting the veganism journey. Your family will thank you for the delicious meals you are serving. Your taste buds will thank you, too.

ROOT VEGETABLE DAL

If you love light foods to consume for lunch, I recommend you try this remarkably flavorsome vegan, gluten-free root vegetable dal loaded with nutrients to kick-start your weight loss journey.

Nutritional information for one serving:

- Total Calories: 306
- Protein: 12 grams
- Fat: 19 grams
- Fiber: 7 grams
- Carbohydrates: 28 grams

Ingredients:

- 1 cup of red split lentils, rinsed
- 1 cup of finely diced root vegetables of your choice, like celery, beets and carrots
- 1 small onion, finely diced

- 1 cup of grape or cherry tomatoes, halved
- 4 cloves of minced garlic
- 2-inch piece of fresh ginger, peeled and minced
- 1 teaspoon of ground turmeric
- Pinch of dried chili flakes
- 3 1/2 cups of filtered water
- Salt and pepper to taste
- 2 tablespoons of virgin coconut oil
- 1/2 teaspoon of cumin seeds
- 1/2 teaspoon of coriander seeds
- 1/2 teaspoon of mustard seeds
- 1/3 cup of chopped fresh cilantro for garnish
- Lemon wedges for serving

Method:

1. The initial step is to prepare a medium soup pot and add in the rinsed lentils, vegetables, diced root, diced onion, tomatoes, garlic, chili flakes, turmeric and ginger. Once all in, pour the water into the pot and stir everything well.

2. The following step is to place the soup pot over medium heat. Bring to a gentle boil and then simmer for about forty minutes as whisking often. In the last ten minutes of cooking, whisk the dal vigorously to encourage separation and break-down of the lentils. Season the meal with salt and pepper.

3. The next step is to heat the coconut oil in a small sauté pan placed over medium heat. Then, add in the coriander seeds, cumin seeds and mustard seeds. Once the seeds are popping and fragrant, remove the pot from the heat.

4. The next step is to gently spoon the toasted spice oil on top of the dal. It can be lightly stirred as well. Garnish the dal with the chopped cilantro, serve with lemon wedges and enjoy.

VEGAN SKILLET ENCHILADAS

This is a very simple vegan, gluten-free lunch recipe you can prepare in under thirty minutes making it a perfect dish on those busy days when you have a lot of errands to run and not much to put into meal preparation.

Nutritional information for one serving:

- Total Calories: 309
- Protein: 12.1 grams
- Fat: 7.9 grams
- Fiber: 6.5 grams
- Carbohydrates: 37 grams

Ingredients:

- 2 tablespoons of oil, divided
- 10 small corn tortillas cut into thin strips
- 1/2 large red onion diced

- 2-3 cloves of minced garlic
- 1 small butternut squash peeled and cut into 1/2-inch cubes
- 1 1/2 teaspoon of chili powder
- 1/2 teaspoon of cumin
- 1/2 teaspoon of paprika
- 1/2 teaspoon of salt
- 1 can of black beans
- 1/2 cup of canned or frozen corn
- 1 cup of crushed tomatoes
- 10 oz. of enchiladas sauce
- 4 large kale leaves, chopped
- Salt and pepper to taste
- Several sprigs of chopped cilantro
- 1 jalapeno, diced
- 2 green onions, diced
- 1 avocado

Method:

1. The initial step is to prepare a large, cast iron skillet and heat one tablespoon of oil. Once done, add in the tortilla strips and cook for about five minutes, stirring often. Transfer to a paper towel when done cooking.

2. The next step is to add the remaining amount of oil and the onion and sauté for about five minutes, stirring occasionally, until onions are fragrant and translucent. Once done, add in the garlic and sauté for thirty more seconds.

3. Then, add the chili powder, butternut squash, cumin, salt and paprika. Stir well to coat evenly. Reduce heat to low and cover the pot. Cook until the butternut squash is tender. This will take about five minutes.

4. The following step is to add the corn, black beans, tomatoes, kale and enchilada sauce. Cook for an additional three minutes until the kale is wilted. Once done, season with salt and pepper.

5. The next step is to stir in corn tortillas and bring to a gentle simmer and cook for about ten minutes until the liquid has boiled down.

6. Then, remove enchiladas from heat and let set for ten additional minutes before you serve the meal.

7. Once done, serve it with cilantro, green onions and jalapeno.

CAULIFLOWER AND OYSTER MUSHROOM TACOS

These amazingly tasty cauliflower and oyster mushroom tacos are something that you can prepare in almost no time. This dish is loaded with nutrients, so your weight loss progress can easily continue without any distractions.

Nutritional information for one serving:

- Total Calories: 340
- Protein: 9 grams
- Fat: 16 grams
- Fiber: 11 grams
- Carbohydrates: 45 grams

Ingredients:

- 1 head cauliflower cut into small florets, six to eight cups
- 4 tablespoons of olive oil
- 1 tablespoon of chili powder
- 1 tablespoon of smoked paprika
- 1 teaspoon of ground coriander
- 1/2 teaspoon of ground cumin
- Pinch of red pepper flakes
- Salt and pepper
- 1 cup of thinly sliced Spanish or Vidalia onion
- 1 large or 2 small poblano chilis, sliced
- 1/2 cup of chopped red bell pepper
- 1 clove or minced garlic
- 6 oz. of oyster mushrooms, thinly sliced
- 2 teaspoons of freshly squeezed lime juice
- 8 crisp corn tortillas
- 1/2 cup of chopped fresh cilantro for garnish

Method:

1. The initial step is to preheat the oven to 425 degrees. Then, prepare a large bowl and toss the cauliflower florets with two tablespoons of the olive oil until evenly coated.

2. The next step is to sprinkle the coriander, chili powder, paprika, red pepper flakes, cumin and a generous pinch of salt. Toss the bowl until the cauliflower is evenly coated. Then, spread the mixture on a rimmed baking sheet and bake for at least twenty minutes.

3. Then, heat the remaining two tablespoons of olive oil in a large skillet placed over medium heat. Then, add in the poblano, onion and red bell pepper and sauté until the onion is a bit golden and tender.

4. Once done, add the garlic and sauté for an additional minute. Then, stir in the mushrooms and season with salt and pepper. Cook until the mushrooms are crispy and tender that will take about five minutes.

5. Remove the pot from the heat and stir in the lime juice. Adjust the seasoning, if needed.

6. For each taco, put 1/4 cup of the mushroom mixture in a tortilla. Top them with some of the roasted cauliflower and add a tablespoonful of fresh cilantro. Serve and enjoy.

EGGPLANT CHICKPEA CURRY

This delicious meal can help boost your immune system and prevent disease, aid in healthy digestion, prevent anemia, aid in heart health and much more all thanks to the delicious, yet healthy eggplant.

Nutritional information for one serving:

- Total Calories: 178
- Protein: 6 grams
- Fat: 6 grams
- Fiber: 7 grams
- Carbohydrates: 27 grams

Ingredients:

- 1 tablespoon of coconut oil
- 1 medium onion, thinly sliced
- 3-4 cloves of minced garlic

- 1 tablespoon of fresh ginger, minced
- 1 tablespoon of curry powder
- 1 teaspoon of cumin
- 1/2 teaspoon of turmeric
- 1/4 teaspoon of cayenne pepper
- 1/2 teaspoon of salt
- 1 medium eggplant, chopped into one-inch cubes
- 4 cups of chickpeas, drained and rinsed
- 1 1/2 cup of vegetable broth
- 1/4 fresh cilantro for garnish
- 1 cup of gluten-free uncooked rice

Method:

1. Start by cooking the gluten-free rice according to the package instructions.

2. Then, heat the oil in a large soup pot placed over medium heat. Then, add in onions and sauté as you stir for about five to seven minutes until onions are translucent and

fragrant. Then, add in ginger and garlic and sauté for another minute.

3. Once done, add in cumin, curry powder, turmeric, salt and cayenne pepper. Continue to stir to evenly coat the garlic onion mixture.

4. The next step is to add tomatoes, eggplant, vegetable broth and chickpeas. Bring to a gentle simmer and cook uncovered for about twenty minutes until eggplant and tomatoes are well cooked and about 1/2 of the liquid has been absorbed.

5. Serve the meal over gluten-free rice and some fresh cilantro.

RED LENTIL CURRY SOUP

This tasty vegan, gluten-free red lentil curry soup will most certainly keep you pleasantly full and satisfied during the day. Make sure you prepare plenty of this soup, as your family will ask for more due to its amazing flavor.

Nutritional information for one serving:

- Total Calories: 140
- Protein: 5 grams
- Fat: 6 grams
- Fiber: 5 grams
- Carbohydrates: 20 grams

Ingredients:

- 1 tablespoon of coconut oil
- 1 small yellow onion, diced
- 3-4 cloves of minced garlic

- 1 heaping tablespoon of fresh ginger, peeled and minced
- 1 small red bell pepper, diced
- 1 tablespoon of curry powder
- 1 teaspoon of cumin
- 1/2 teaspoon of turmeric
- 1/8 teaspoon of cayenne pepper
- 2 small sweet potatoes, diced
- 1 1/2 cup of red lentils, rinsed
- 6 cups of vegetable broth
- 1/2 teaspoon of salt or 1/8 teaspoon of pepper to taste
- For topping 2-4 tablespoons of fresh cilantro, chopped
- 1 small avocado, diced
- Fresh lime juice, optional

Method:

1. The initial step is to prepare a large soup pot placed over medium to high heat and heat the coconut oil. Then, add diced garlic and

onions and sauté for about five minutes until onions are translucent and fragrant.

2. The following step is to stir in ginger and sauté for another thirty seconds. Then, add in red bell pepper, cumin, cayenne pepper, curry powder and turmeric. Stir well in to coat the vegetables evenly and then sauté for five more minutes stirring often.

3. While peppers and onions are sautéing, peel and chop the sweet potatoes. Then, add them to the pepper-onion mixture along with the vegetable broth and lentils. Then, bring to a gentle boil.

4. Once done, reduce heat to a gentle simmer.

5. Cook the meal uncovered for about twenty minutes stirring often until potatoes are soft and lentils are broken down. Once done, remove the pot from heat.

6. Using an immersion blender, puree the soup until creamy and smooth. Serve it immediately with preferred toppings. You may also store it in an airtight container in the refrigerator for up to five days.

MEDITERRANEAN LENTILS AND RICE

This Mediterranean lentils and rice recipe is perfect for body cleansing. It is loaded with nutrients to keep you full and satisfied during the day. Prepare it for lunch in less than thirty minutes and enjoy immediately.

Nutritional information for one serving:

- Total Calories: 331
- Protein: 23 grams
- Fat: 8 grams
- Fiber: 13 grams
- Carbohydrates: 41 grams

Ingredients:

- 1/2 cup of uncooked basmati rice, gluten-free
- 1/2 cup of uncooked brown lentils, rinsed

- 1 batch of tomato-cucumber salad
- 1/2 cup of homemade or store-bought hummus
- 1/2 small cucumber, thinly sliced
- 4-6 thinly sliced radishes
- 1 small avocado, sliced
- 1/4 cup of Kalamata olives, pitted and halved, optional
- For tomato-cucumber salad: 1 small cucumber
- 2 cups of cherry tomatoes, quartered
- 4 green onions, sliced
- 1 cup of chopped parsley
- Juice of 1 small lemon
- To taste salt and pepper

Method:

1. Start with combining lentils and rice in a medium pot with around 2 1/4 cups of water. Then, bring the water to a gentle boil and reduce heat to let it simmer until the water

has evaporated and the lentils and rice are cooked through.

2. In the meantime, while the lentils and rice are cooking, prepare the vegetables in a large salad bowl and set aside.

3. Prepare a small bowl and combine the listed ingredients to make the tomato-cucumber salad and refrigerate it until you are ready to serve it.

4. Once the lentils and rice are cooked, divide the mixture into four serving plates or bowls. Top them with the tomato-cucumber salad and add radishes, cucumbers, olives and avocado on top of hummus. Serve immediately and enjoy.

QUINOA FALAFEL WITH AVOCADO TAHINI DRESSING

If you love falafel, you will most certainly love this delicious vegan, gluten-free quinoa falafel with tasty avocado tahini dressing loaded with nutrients. Your taste buds will thank you, so make sure you prepare this meal as soon as you can.

Nutritional information for one serving:

- Total Calories: 190
- Protein: 7 grams
- Fat: 10 grams
- Fiber: 3 grams
- Carbohydrates: 17 grams

Ingredients:

- 18 fl. oz. of can chickpeas, rinsed and drained
- Vegetable oil
- 1 medium onion, chopped
- 1 clove of minced garlic
- 1/3 cup of cooked quinoa
- 2 tablespoons of cilantro, fresh coriander
- 1 tablespoon of ground cumin
- 1/4 teaspoon of salt
- 1/4 teaspoon of pepper
- 2 vegan eggs like Ener-G Egg Replacer
- For avocado tahini dressing: 1 ripe avocado
- 1/4 cup of tahini
- 1 tablespoon of fresh lime juice, about 1/2 lime
- 2 tablespoons of cilantro
- 1/2 cup of water

Method:

1. The initial step is to blend all ingredients for dressing using a food processor or blender. Once done, set aside.
2. The next step is to pulse the chickpeas in the food processor until no more whole chickpeas are visible. Then heat one tablespoon of vegetable oil in a frying pan placed over medium heat and fry the garlic and onions until soft.

3. The following step is to combine onion mixture, chickpeas, cilantro, salt, pepper, quinoa, cumin and vegan egg mixture.

4. Once done, form the mixture into twelve balls. Then, heat a couple tablespoons of vegetable oil in the frying pan placed over medium heat. Once done, add the falafel patties and cook for about three minutes on each side until lightly browned.

5. Serve the falafel balls with dressing and enjoy.

ZUCCHINI NOODLES WITH PISTACHIO PESTO

You will absolutely love this simple, yet tasty lunch recipe that you can prepare in just twenty minutes making this a perfect lunch dish for those days when you are extra busy.

Nutritional information for one serving:

- Total Calories: 281
- Protein: 12 grams
- Fat: 16 grams
- Fiber: 0.4 grams
- Carbohydrates: 22 grams

Ingredients:

- 5-6 zucchini, peeled and thinly sliced
- 1 clove of garlic

- 1/2 cup plus 3 tablespoons of shelled pistachios
- 1-2 tablespoons of lemon juice
- Zest of one lemon
- 1/4 teaspoon of salt
- 2 cups of parsley or 1 cup of cilantro and 1 cup of parsley
- 1/2 cup of olive oil

Method:

1. The initial step is to prepare the zucchini in a large salad bowl.

2. Once done, combine the garlic, lemon juice, 1/2 cup of pistachios, lemon zest, parsley and salt in the food processor and pulse five times until everything is integrated.

3. Then, add the olive oil as the food processor is running and process until all ingredients are well combined.

4. Then, mix the zucchini with the pistachio pesto.

5. To serve the meal, chop the remaining pistachios and sprinkle them over the top.

CHAPTER 3: DINNER RECIPES

Going vegan and gluten-free can greatly improve a person's overall health and help support their general well-being. Almost immediately after deciding to start following a vegan diet, you will notice positive changes in your body as well as in your mind. You start feeling more energized; always one step closer to your ideal weight.

Despite the fact you must avoid certain foods, you can enjoy delicious meals loaded with nutrients that will help you boost your weight loss progress. In the following section of the book, you are going to learn simple, yet tasty dinner recipes you can prepare in less than thirty minutes. As you delight your taste buds with these delectable recipes, be sure to remember which one your family liked the best, so you can prepare more the next time you make it.

FIG SPINACH SALAD WITH BALSAMIC VINAIGRETTE

If you enjoy salads, you will love this vegan, gluten-free fig, spinach salad loaded with tasty balsamic vinaigrette. It is perfect for a dinner meal you share with your family members. This easy meal can be put together and be on your table in less than twenty minutes.

Nutritional information for one serving:

- Total Calories: 207
- Protein: 2.7 grams
- Fat: 9.9 grams
- Fiber: 6.6 grams
- Carbohydrates: 32.2 grams

Ingredients:

- 2 large handfuls of fresh spinach
- 4 figs cut in half
- 1 small avocado, pitted and sliced
- 1/3 cup of walnuts
- 1/4 cup of red onions, chopped
- For balsamic vinaigrette: 1/2 cup of extra-virgin olive oil
- 1/4 cup of balsamic vinegar
- 1-2 cloves of garlic minced
- 1 tablespoon of Dijon mustard
- 1 teaspoon of maple syrup
- Salt and pepper to taste

Method:

1. The initial step is to prepare a small blender and combine the ingredients listed for the balsamic vinaigrette. Once done, set the bowl aside.

2. The next step is to roast the walnuts at 400 degrees for five to seven minutes until they turn brown. Remove the pan from heat and let cool.

3. Then, divide spinach between two serving plates and top with the remaining salad ingredients. Serve the salad immediately with balsamic vinaigrette and enjoy.

RICE, BEAN AND KALE BOWL WITH LEMON-DILL TAHINI

Going vegan and gluten-free is the most efficient and way to turn to a healthier lifestyle. You can enjoy this delicious rice, bean and kale bowl filled with lemon-dill tahini for the perfect finish of every day.

Nutritional information for one serving:

- Total Calories: 146
- Protein: 2 grams
- Fat: 6.8 grams
- Fiber: 0.7 grams
- Carbohydrates: 4 grams

Ingredients:

- 1 can of black beans
- 1 cup of hummus or tahini
- 1/2 cup of lemon juice
- 1 tablespoon of fresh dill
- 1 cup of cooked brown rice, gluten-free
- 1 bunch of kale, steamed
- 1 teaspoon of vegan Parmesan, optional

Method:

1. The initial step is to heat the black beans in a medium saucepan placed over medium heat.

2. The following step is to mix the lemon juice, tahini and dill together in a small container.

3. Whisk until the mixture reaches the consistency that resembles dressing.

4. The next step is to layer the black beans, cooked brown rice and steamed kale in a

large bowl and top with the tasty tahini dressing. You may sprinkle some vegan Parmesan on top and enjoy.

CURRIED LENTILS WITH CARROTS AND CHICKPEAS

If you need a simple, no-fuss dinner for your weeknight meals, consider preparing this easy to make curried lentils with carrots and chickpeas recipe that is high in protein, soy free, and dairy free.

Nutritional information for one serving:

- Total Calories: 190
- Protein: 18 grams
- Fat: 2 grams
- Fiber: 16 grams
- Carbohydrates: 36 grams

Ingredients:

- A good handful of arugula or any other leafy green of your choice, per serving plate
- 2 cups of red lentils, rinsed and cooked in four cups of water
- 1 cup of cooked chickpeas
- 1 big carrot, cut into little chunks
- 1 clove of minced garlic
- 1/2 onion, cut in small pieces
- 2 teaspoons of curry powder
- A dash of turmeric, optional
- Several dashes of dried ginger or grate 1/2 teaspoon of fresh ginger
- 1 teaspoon of coconut oil
- 1 tablespoon of parsley
- For topping almonds

Method:

1. The initial step is to cook the lentils in the four cups of water.

2. In the meantime, heat the coconut oil in a saucepan and add the onion. Once the onions become soft, add the carrot chunks or slices.

3. The following step is to add the chickpeas. Stir and add the dried spices and finish with the garlic.

4. Once the lentils are cooked through which will take about eight minutes, add them to the other mixture as well. Once done, serve the salad on a serving plate with greens you prefer and enjoy.

MEXICAN TOFU SCRAMBLE

If you love quick and easy to make recipes that are incredibly appetizing, I suggest you prepare this Mexican tofu scramble. It is a perfect dinner recipe that you can prepare quickly that will suit both you and your family's wishes as a satisfying meal.

Nutritional information for one serving:

- Total Calories: 178
- Protein: 15 grams
- Fat: 9 grams
- Fiber: 5 grams
- Carbohydrates: 12 grams

Ingredients:

- 8 oz. of extra firm tofu
- 2 tablespoons of nutritional yeast
- 1/4 teaspoon of salt

- Juice of 1/2 lemon
- 1-2 tablespoons of cooking oil
- 1/2 red onion, chopped
- 1/2 red bell pepper, chopped
- 2-3 cloves of garlic, minced
- 1 jalapeno pepper, seeded and minced
- 1/2 cup of corn
- 3/4 cup of Pico de Gallo
- For topping: Fresh lime
- Cilantro
- Avocado

Method:

1. Start with preparing a small bowl where you crumble tofu to the texture of scrambled eggs. Then, add nutritional yeast, lemon juice and salt and set aside.

2. The next step is to prepare a large skillet and heat oil placed over medium heat. Once heated, add onions and sauté for about five minutes. Stir often.

3. The next step is to add garlic, bell pepper and jalapeno pepper and sauté for another five minutes until the bell pepper is soft.

4. The following step is to stir in crumbled tofu and corn. Heat ingredients all the way through as you stir frequently.

5. Remove the pot from the heat and stir in Pico de Gallo. Once done, serve meal immediately with toppings of your choice and enjoy.

THAI QUINOA SALAD WITH SESAME PEANUT SAUCE

This is an extraordinarily delightful dinner recipe you will love from the very first moment you taste it. This Thai quinoa salad loaded with sesame peanut sauce is a perfect choice for those people who like light dinners that burst with flavor.

Nutritional information for one serving:

- Total Calories: 260
- Protein: 8.6 grams
- Fat: 13.5 grams
- Fiber: 4.3 grams
- Carbohydrates: 27.7 grams

Ingredients:

- 1 bag of Success tri-Color Quinoa
- 2 cups of red cabbage, shredded
- 1 1/2 cups of broccoli florets, chopped
- 1/2 large red bell pepper, thinly sliced
- 1 large carrot, chopped
- 3 green onions, chopped
- 1/4 cup of cilantro
- 1 batch of sesame peanut sauce
- 1/4 cup of roasted peanuts
- For sesame peanut sauce: 1/4 cup of natural peanut butter
- 2 tablespoons of sesame oil
- 2 tablespoons of soy sauce
- 1 tablespoon of rice vinegar
- 2 tablespoons of garlic, minced
- 1 teaspoon of maple syrup

Method:

1. The initial step is to prepare the Success Quinoa according to the package

instructions. In the meantime, while the quinoa is boiling, chop the bell peppers, cabbage, carrots, green onions, broccoli and cilantro and set aside.

2. The next step is to combine all ingredients listed for the peanut sauce in a small blender. Blend until the mixture is smooth and creamy.

3. Then, with a slotted spoon or tongs, remove the quinoa from boiling water. Cut open the bag and let it cool for at least ten minutes.

4. Then, place the quinoa in a large salad bowl and add already prepared vegetables. Toss with peanut sauce and peanuts.

5. Serve salad immediately or store it in an airtight container in the refrigerator for up to three days.

VEGGIE AND BEAN BURGERS

Following a vegan diet can be extremely enjoyable especially when you get to relish these delicious vegan, gluten-free burgers made of veggies and beans. You will not be able to tell the difference from real burgers.

Nutritional information for one serving:

- Total Calories: 247
- Protein: 8 grams
- Fat: 9 grams
- Fiber: 6 grams
- Carbohydrates: 36 grams

Ingredients:

- 1 1/2 cups of cooked chickpeas or beans of your choice
- 2 tablespoons of olive oil

- 2 cloves of minced garlic
- 1 small white onion, diced
- 2 small carrots, diced
- 1/2 cup of gluten-free flour
- 1 flax egg: One flax egg you can make by combining one tablespoon of ground flaxseed mixed with three tablespoons of water.
- 2 tablespoons of chopped fresh herbs
- 1 teaspoon of cumin
- 1/2 teaspoon of sea salt

Method:

1. Start with placing olive oil in a medium skillet over low to medium heat. Once heated, add garlic, onion and carrots and cook for about five to ten minutes until oils are fragrant and vegetables are soft.

2. The next step is to combine all ingredients in a food processor and pulse until they are all

well combined. Once done, form the mixture into four round patties.

3. Then, cook in a large skillet, which has been lightly coated with olive oil placed over medium heat. This will take about five minutes per each side. Serve warm and enjoy.

CHICKPEA CRUST PIZZA

As soon as you make this delightfully tasty vegan, gluten-free chickpea crust pizza you are going to love it. The meal is loaded with awesome flavors that will satisfy your taste buds.

Nutritional information for one serving:

- Total Calories: 180
- Protein: 8 grams
- Fat: 7 grams
- Fiber: 4 grams
- Carbohydrates: 23 grams

Ingredients:

- 2 cups of chickpea flour
- 1 cup of water
- 2 teaspoons of olive oil
- Dash of salt

- 1/2 cup of marinara or pizza sauce
- Handful of shredded kale
- 1 teaspoon of olive oil
- 1/2 cup of vegan cheese, you may use Daiya mozzarella

Method:

1. The initial step is to preheat the oven to 375 degrees. Then, line a baking sheet with parchment paper.

2. The following step is to prepare a medium bowl and stir together water, flour, two teaspoons of olive oil, salt and whisk until all ingredients are well combined.

3. To prepare pizza crust, spread the mixture out in a circular shape. You may make several smaller pizza crusts as well.

4. Bake the pizza crust in the oven for about fifteen to twenty minutes until crust edges turn slightly crispy.

5. In the meantime, while the crust bakes, toss kale in a small salad bowl with one teaspoon of olive oil.

6. The next step is to remove crust from the oven. Flip parchment paper and crust upside down on the baking sheet. Then, gently pull the baking sheet away from the pizza crust.

7. The following step is to spread sauce over pizza crust. Then, layer kale over sauce and sprinkle with vegan cheese. Bake in the oven five to seven minutes. Once done, slice the pizza and enjoy right away.

ENCHILADAS VERDE

You will probably fall in love with this astoundingly scrumptious dinner meal from the very first moment you taste it. These tasty enchiladas Verde are one of the simplest, yet most delicious meals you can prepare for dinner and in less than forty-five minutes.

Nutritional information for one serving:

- Total Calories: 390
- Protein: 16 grams
- Fat: 17 grams
- Fiber: 7 grams
- Carbohydrates: 38 grams

Ingredients:

- For cashew cream: 1/2 cup of water
- 1 cup of cashews

- 2 teaspoons of apple cider vinegar
- 1 serrano pepper roasted, optional
- Juice of 1 lemon
- 1 teaspoon of agave or maple syrup
- Salt to taste
- For enchiladas: 1/2 batch of Salsa Verde or store bought green salsa
- 10 corn tortillas
- 1 tablespoon of olive oil
- 1 15 oz. can of corn
- 3 small zucchinis
- 1/2 white onion, sliced
- 5-6 cloves of garlic
- 4 cups of loosely packed kale, thinly chopped
- 1 15 oz. can of black beans
- Salt and pepper to taste
- For topping: 1 avocado
- 1 handful of cilantro
- 2-3 green onions

Method:

1. To make the cashew cream, place all listed ingredients in a high-powered blender and blend until smooth. Once completed, place the mixture into the refrigerator until you want to use it. If you do not have a high-powered blender, you can soak the cashews for at least four hours prior to use.

2. The next step is to make the Salsa Verde. Preheat the oven to broil; place husked tomatillos, garlic and poblanos on a baking sheet. Then, drizzle with olive oil and broil for at least five minutes until vegetables are tender.

3. Then, flip peppers and tomatillos and broil for another five minutes. Remove the pan from oven and let it cool for ten minutes.

4. Then, place the tomatillos, garlic and peppers in a food processor with cilantro,

onion, lime juice and cumin. Pulse until all vegetables are broken down. Then, salt and pepper to taste.

5. Once you have made the Salsa Verde sauce, prepare enchiladas. Preheat the oven to 350 degrees. Then, slice zucchini in 1/2-inch pieces and mix them with garlic, corn and onions. Then, drizzle one tablespoon of olive oil over vegetables and spread evenly on the baking sheet. Roast for about twenty minutes and stir often until vegetables are fragrant.

6. The next step is to prepare a large skillet and sauté black beans and kale until kale has wilted a bit. Then, add the roasted vegetables mixture to the bean-kale mixture along with 1/2 cup of salsa Verde.

7. Then, soften the corn tortillas to make them pliable. To do this, wrap them in a slightly damp paper towel or damp cloth and

microwave them for about thirty seconds until steaming. This steam will soften the corn tortillas, so they can be rolled.

8. The next step is to place 1/2 cup of green salsa on bottom of an 8x12 baking dish. Then, put about 1/4 cup of filling in each tortilla and gently roll up. Repeat this process until all tortillas are gone and there is no more filling.

9. Bake for about forty-five minutes until the filling starts to bubble. Remove the pan from the oven and let it cool for at least ten minutes before you serve the meal with toppings of your choice and cashew cream. Enjoy.

CHAPTER 4: SIDES AND SNACKS RECIPES

In the following section of the book, you are going to learn some delicious sides and snacks recipes. They are all vegan, gluten-free recipes and will be of immense help when it comes to boosting your weight loss progress.

I suggest you always make more, as you taste buds will ask for more for sure. Being on a vegan diet does not mean you have to give up on delicious treats. You just focus on consuming snacks that are vegan-gluten-free, but as tasty as any other regular treat. Inside this book, you are given many delicious options so there shouldn't be any disruption to your weight loss progress.

CHICKPEA SALAD

If you love salads, you will most certainly love this amazingly tasty vegan gluten-free chickpea salad you can prepare under fifteen minutes and serve with almost any main dish you have on your table.

Nutritional information for one serving:

- Total Calories: 190
- Protein: 5 grams
- Fat: 9 grams
- Fiber: 0.2 grams
- Carbohydrates: 21 grams

Ingredients:

- 15 oz. of can chickpeas, drained and rinsed
- 2 stalks of celery, chopped finely
- 3 green onions, thinly sliced
- 1/4 cup of finely chopped dill pickle

- 1/4 cup of finely chopped red bell pepper
- 3 tablespoons of store-bought or homemade vegan mayonnaise
- 1 clove of minced garlic
- 1 1/2 teaspoons of yellow mustard
- 2 teaspoons of fresh dill, optional
- 1 1/2 to 3 teaspoons of fresh melon juice to taste
- 1/4 teaspoon of fine sea salt to taste
- Fresh ground black pepper

Method:

1. The initial step is to prepare a large salad bowl and mash the chickpeas with a potato masher until the chickpeas are flaked in texture.

2. The next step is to stir in the celery, pickles, bell peppers, green onions, garlic and mayonnaise until all ingredients are well combined.

3. Then, stir in the dill, mustard and season with the lemon juice, salt and pepper. Make sure you adjust the quantities to taste.

4. Serve the salad with toasted gluten-free bread, crackers, wraps or on top of a leafy green salad. You may enjoy it all on its own as well. If you want a soy-free version of this salad, just use soy-free vegan mayonnaise.

ZUCCHINI SQUARES

You are going to absolutely love these surprisingly mouthwatering zucchini squares that make a perfect vegan, gluten-free snack you can eat at any time during the day without worrying about calories.

Nutritional information for one serving:

- Total Calories: 153
- Protein: 1.8 grams
- Fat: 4.9 grams
- Fiber: 0.5 grams
- Carbohydrates: 28.7 grams

Ingredients:

- 1/4 cup of melted allergy-friendly shortening
- 1 cup of shredded zucchini, measured with the liquid already pressed out

- 1 flax egg: 1 tablespoon of flax meal plus 3 tablespoons of warm water
- 2 tablespoons of water or your favorite dairy-free milk substitute
- 1 teaspoon of vanilla extract
- 1 1/2 cup of Enjoy Life Foods All-Purpose Flour Mix
- 1/2 cup of quinoa flakes
- 1/2 cup of cooked white quinoa
- 1 teaspoon of guar gum or 1/2 teaspoons of xanthan gum
- 1 teaspoon of baking soda
- 1/2 teaspoon of salt
- 1/4 teaspoon of ground cinnamon
- 1/2 cup of Enjoy Life Foods Mini Chips
- Optional topping 1/4 cup of toasted pumpkin seeds
- 1/4 cup of raw amaranth
- 1/4 cup of Enjoy Life Foods Mini Chips

Method:

1. The initial step is to preheat the oven to 350 degrees. Then, line a 9x9 baking sheet with parchment paper and set aside.

2. The next step is to prepare a large mixing bowl and mix together the shortening, flax egg, water, zucchini and vanilla. Make sure to whisk until all ingredients are well blended.

3. Use a separate bowl and whisk the remaining ingredients except those for toppings, from the Mini Chips through the All-Purpose Flour.

4. Then, pour the flour mixture into the shortening mixture and stir until all ingredients are well combined. This will take around two minutes. Then, pour the mixture into the already prepared baking pan and sprinkle toppings, if using.

5. Bake for about fifteen minutes, rotate the dish and bake for another fifteen minutes until a toothpick inserted into the center of the dish comes clean.

6. Cool the meal the in pan. Cut it into smaller squares. Serve and enjoy.

LOW-CARB PIZZA STICKS

If you want to make simple, yet tasty snacks that your entire family can enjoy, I suggest you prepare these amazingly delicious, low-carb pizza sticks. Make sure you make a bunch of them, as your family will most certainly ask for more.

Nutritional information for one serving:

- Total Calories: 40
- Protein: 4 grams
- Fat: 2 grams
- Fiber: 1 grams
- Carbohydrates: 2 grams

Ingredients:

- 1 block of extra firm tofu
- 1/4 cup plus 1 tablespoon of tomato sauce

- 2 tablespoons plus 2 teaspoons of nutritional yeast
- Several pinches of dried basil

Method:

1. The initial step is to drain tofu by wrapping the block of tofu in a paper towel. Then, place a cutting board on top of that block of tofu. Make sure you apply even pressure to the top of every block by placing a cookbook or something else you have of equal weight on top of the cutting board. Once done, leave the tofu to drain for about fifteen minutes.

2. In the meantime, while the tofu is draining, preheat the oven to 425 degrees and line a baking sheet with parchment paper.

3. The next step is to cut the tofu into 16 thin pieces and place them on a baking sheet. Spread one teaspoon of marinara sauce on every pizza stick.

4. Sprinkle the pizza sticks with 1/2 teaspoon of nutritional yeast. In addition, sprinkle basil over the pizza sticks to taste.

5. Bake for about thirty minutes, serve and enjoy.

SPICY BUFFALO CAULIFLOWER WINGS

You are going to absolutely love this incredibly simple, yet highly nutritious side dish you can serve with various main meals. These spicy Buffalo cauliflower wings make a perfect complement to both lunch and dinner meals you are going to enjoy.

Nutritional information for one serving:

- Total Calories: 221
- Protein: 14 grams
- Fat: 12 grams
- Fiber: 0.2 grams
- Carbohydrates: 15 grams

Ingredients:

- 1 cup of water or soy milk
- 1 cup of flour, gluten-free
- 2 teaspoons of garlic powder
- 1 head of cauliflower, chopped into small pieces
- 1 cup of buffalo or hot sauce
- 1 tablespoon of vegetable oil or melted vegan butter

Method:

1. The initial step is to preheat the oven to 450 degrees. Then, combine the soy milk or water, garlic powder and flour in a large bowl and stir until all ingredients are well combined.

2. The next step is to coat the cauliflower pieces with the flour mixture and place it in a shallow baking dish.

3. Bake for about eighteen minutes.

4. In the meantime, while the cauliflower is baking, combine olive oil or margarine with the buffalo sauce in a small bowl.

5. Then, pour the hot sauce mixture over the baked cauliflower pieces and continue baking for an additional five to eight minutes.

6. Once done, serve the cauliflower wings alongside celery sticks and vegan blue cheese dressing.

MISO SESAME KALE BOWL-ED OVER

This remarkably delightful miso sesame kale bowl-ed over will probably become your favorite side dish. You can serve it with almost any lunch and dinner meal, so make sure you try it as soon as possible.

Nutritional information for one serving:

- Total Calories: 474
- Protein: 18 grams
- Fat: 20 grams
- Fiber: 7 grams
- Carbohydrates: 62 grams

Ingredients:

- For salad: 4 cups of chopped raw kale
- 1 cup of prepared sauerkraut, milder flavored recommended

- 1/4 cup of toasted sesame seeds
- 2 cups of cooked wild brown or brown gluten-free rice mixture
- For sauce: 1/4 cup of water
- 1 tablespoon of gluten-free tamari sauce or Braggs
- 2 tablespoons of white miso paste
- 2 tablespoons of tahini
- 1/2 teaspoon of ginger

Method:

1. Start with preparing the non-stock pan by placing it over medium to high heat to brown the sesame seeds. Once done, remove the seeds to a bowl.

2. Using the same pan, add kale as you stir often until kale is wilted. Then, move kale to one side of the pan and place sauerkraut on the other side. Turn down heat to low, cover with lid, and allow sauerkraut to warm up.

3. To prepare sauce, add water, miso, tahini, Braggs and ginger to a blender or food processor and mix thoroughly until the mixture becomes smooth and creamy.

4. Then, spoon cooked rice into a bowl, top with sauerkraut and kale. Then, pour on miso sauce to taste. Make sure you top the mixture by sprinkling on some toasted sesame seeds. Serve and enjoy.

GREEN POWER BOWL

If crispy roasted potatoes, finely chopped collard greens and tasty broccoli sound good to you, then you are going to love this low in calories, easy to prepare, green power bowl loaded with nutrients.

Nutritional information for one serving:

- Total Calories: 95
- Protein: 3 grams
- Fat: 3.5 grams
- Fiber: 3 grams
- Carbohydrates: 6 grams

Ingredients:

- 5 large collard green leaves
- 1 cup of diced potatoes
- 1 cup of chopped broccoli
- 1/4 teaspoon of paprika powder

- 1/4 teaspoon of salt
- 1/8 teaspoon of garlic powder
- 1/2 teaspoon of dried rosemary

Method:

1. The initial step is to wash and dice the potatoes.

2. Then, prepare a large pan and heat the coconut oil. Then toss in the diced potatoes when the oil is hot. Season with paprika powder, garlic powder, salt and dried rosemary. Then, put the lid on and roast the potatoes placed over medium to high heat for about five to ten minutes until the potatoes are soft. Make sure you stir often.

3. The next step is to add in the chopped broccoli and let it roast for another five minutes until tender.

4. The following step is to wash the collard greens and remove stems. Then, roll it up, cut into thin slices, and add them to the pan.

5. Season with salt and let it roast on medium heat for about five minutes. Make sure the lid is on. Stir everything together thoroughly and add more salt to taste. You may turn the heat to high towards the end if the potatoes are not brown and crispy.

6. Divide the mixture between two serving plates and enjoy.

RED LENTIL AND AMARANTH PROTEIN PATTIES

If you are looking for a wonderfully appetizing snack you can prepare almost in no time, consider making these surprisingly delectable red lentil and amaranth protein patties that will make your taste buds happy.

Nutritional information for one serving:

- Total Calories: 290
- Protein: 13 grams
- Fat: 10 grams
- Fiber: 14 grams
- Carbohydrates: 41 grams

Ingredients:

- For protein patties: 1/2 cup of amaranth, uncooked
- 1/2 cup of red lentils, uncooked
- 2 cups of water
- 1 medium Russet potato, grated
- 1 small onion, chopped
- 2 cloves or chopped garlic
- 1/2 cup of parsley, chopped
- 1 tablespoon of nutritional yeast
- 1 tablespoon of mustard
- 2 tablespoons of ketchup
- 2 tablespoons of rice flour
- 2 tablespoons of coarse cornmeal
- 1/2 teaspoon of cumin
- 1 teaspoon of paprika
- 1 teaspoon of sea salt
- 1/2 teaspoon of black pepper
- For the spicy avocado mayo: 1 ripe of mashed avocado
- 2 tablespoons of vegan mayonnaise

- 1 teaspoon of balsamic vinegar
- 1 teaspoon of olive oil
- 1 pinch of sea salt
- A pinch of cayenne pepper

Method:

1. The initial step is to preheat the oven to 450 degrees. Then, place one to two tablespoons of high heat oil like canola, grape seed or avocado on the baking sheet and spread evenly.

2. The next step is to prepare a medium pot and place amaranth, two cups of water and lentils. Bring to a gentle boil, cover the pot and reduce to a simmer. Then, let it cook for about ten to fifteen minutes until water has evaporated and lentils and amaranth are cooked. Once done, let it cool.

3. In the meantime, while the amaranth is cooking, grate the potato in a large mixing

bowl. Once done, using your hands squeeze the shredded potatoes over the sink to release excess water. Then, return to bowl and add garlic, chopped onion and parsley. Then, add in cooked lentil amaranth mixture and mix well using your hands. Add spices, mustard, rice flour, ketchup and cornmeal and mix well until all ingredients are well combined.

4. Then, divide mixture to form small patties. Once done, place them on the baking sheet and bake for about ten minutes on each side until they turn to golden brown color.

5. In the meantime, make the homemade avocado mayo. Simply mash avocado in a small bowl using a fork. Then, add rest of listed ingredients and stir well. Once done, serve the protein patties with the avocado mayo on the side as a dipping sauce and enjoy.

BACON FLAVORED ROASTED CHICKPEAS

This tasty and easy to make snack is sure to be one of your favorites as you can have it ready to serve in less than an hour. Make sure you make a bunch of these bacon flavored roasted chickpeas as your taste buds will most certainly ask for more.

Nutritional information for one serving:

- Total Calories: 141
- Protein: 6 grams
- Fat: 4 grams
- Fiber: 5 grams
- Carbohydrates: 3 grams

Ingredients:

- 15 oz. can of chickpeas, drained and rinsed
- 1/2 cup of soy sauce
- 2 tablespoons of tomato paste
- 2 tablespoons of vegan Worcestershire
- 2 tablespoons of maple syrup
- 1 tablespoon of liquid smoke
- 1/8 teaspoon of pepper
- 1 tablespoon of olive oil

Method:

1. Prepare a shallow dish and whisk together the tomato paste, soy sauce, maple syrup, Worcestershire, pepper and liquid smoke. Then, add chickpeas. Make sure they are fully submerged. Marinate them for at least one hour or even better overnight.

2. Then, preheat the oven to 400 degrees and line a sheet pan with a silicone baking mat or parchment paper and set aside.

3. The next step is to drain the chickpeas from the marinade. Then, blot the chickpeas dry. Then, toss with olive oil and 1/4 cup of reserved marinade. Spread it evenly on the baking sheet.

4. Bake for at least thirty-five minutes stirring every ten minutes to allow for even cooking. Make sure to bake until the chickpeas are crunchy and brown. To prevent burning, watch them closely towards the end.

5. Store the roasted chickpeas in an airtight container at room temperature for up to five days and serve them immediately as a side dish.

CHAPTER 5: DESSEERT RECIPES

Losing weight as you follow a vegan and gluten-free lifestyle does not have to be difficult at all especially as you get to enjoy delicious sweet treats made at home by you. In the following section of the book, you are going to learn several wonderful and tasty sweet treats and desserts that you and your family will love from the very first taste.

The recipes listed are very simple using ingredients you probably already have in your kitchen. They are also very nutritious as well as appetizing, so you don't feel cheated while following this healthy lifestyle.

CHOCOLATE CHIP CHEWY BARS

These astonishingly mouthwatering chocolate chip chewy bars will be a great surprise for you and your family members. You can make a bunch of them and save them for later as well. Either way, you are going to enjoy.

Nutritional information for one serving:

- Total Calories: 140
- Protein: 2 grams
- Fat: 9 grams
- Fiber: 4 grams
- Carbohydrates: 14 grams

Ingredients:

- 1/2 cup of packed brown sugar
- 1/3 cup of peanut butter
- 1/4 cup of agave nectar or maple syrup

- 1/4 cup of vegan butter, melted
- 1 cup of quick-cooking oats, gluten-free
- 1/8 cup of sunflower kernels
- 1/8 cup of walnut pieces
- 1/4 cup of dairy-free chocolate chips
- Pinch of salt
- Pinch of cinnamon, optional
- 1 small handful of raisins, optional

Method:

1. The initial step is to preheat the oven to 350 degrees. Then, in a mixing bowl combine the peanut butter, brown sugar, agave and vegan butter. Then, stir in the kernels, oats, walnuts, salt, cinnamon, raisins and chocolate chips. Be sure to cool down the mixture, so the chocolate chips do not melt from the warm butter.

2. The next step is to place the mixture on two to three pieces of aluminum foil over a cookie sheet, so the bars cook evenly.

3. Then, bake for twelve to fifteen minutes until the edges start to turn to light brown. Once done, remove the pan from the oven and let the cookies cool down entirely before you serve them.

COFFEE CREAM BARS

If you are a fan of flavorful, tasty sweet treats like anyone else, you will love these easy to make, yet delicious coffee cream bars you can prepare in less than thirty minutes.

Nutritional information for one serving:

- Total Calories: 189
- Protein: 4 3grams
- Fat: 12.7 grams
- Fiber: 2 grams
- Carbohydrates: 18 grams

Ingredients:

- For crust: 1 cup of raw cashews
- 1 cup of dates
- 2 teaspoons of instant coffee granules

- 2 tablespoons of water, optional in case your crust does not come together
- For filling: 1 14 oz. canned coconut cream
- 2 teaspoons of instant coffee granules
- 3-4 tablespoons of maple syrup
- 2 tablespoons of Kahlua
- For topping: 3 tablespoons of coconut oil, melted
- 3 tablespoons of cacao powder
- 3 tablespoons of maple syrup

Method:

1. The initial step is to place all the crust ingredients in the food processor and pulse until the mixture seems to be coming together and all ingredients are well combined.

2. Using a spatula, press the mixture evenly into the bottom of an 8x8 inch baking pan that was previously lined with unbleached parchment paper.

3. The next step is to blend the filling ingredients in a food processor until smooth. Then, spread them evenly over the crust and freeze until the topping is prepared. Make sure you freeze it for at least forty-five minutes.

4. In order to prepare the topping, use a small bowl, mix all topping ingredients and pour them over the middle layer. Make sure to spread it evenly.

5. Freeze the coffee bars until firm. To serve them, let the bars thaw at room temperature for about fifteen minutes. Once done, cut them and enjoy.

LEMON BLUEBERRY SWIRL CHEESECAKE SQUARES

This is an incredibly flavorsome vegan, gluten-free dessert you will most certainly enjoy. These tasty lemon blueberry swirl cheesecake squares are so easy to make and are perfect for those days when you do not have that much time to spare on preparing desserts.

Nutritional information for one serving:

- Total Calories: 221
- Protein: 2 grams
- Fat: 7.4 grams
- Fiber: 0.8 grams
- Carbohydrates: 31 grams

Ingredients:

- For the filling: 3 cups of organic raw cashews
- 1 1/2 cup of organic lemon juice
- 3/4 cups of organic maple syrup
- 1 1/4 cup of organic coconut oil
- For the crust: 2 cups of organic raw pecans
- 1/4 cup of organic maple syrup
- 2 tablespoons of organic coconut oil
- 1/2 teaspoon of organic vanilla bean powder
- For the swirl: 1 cup of organic blueberries
- 1 tablespoon of organic maple syrup
- 1 tablespoon of organic coconut oil

Method:

1. The initial step is to add all ingredients listed for the crust in a food processor and process until the mixture has a crumbly, sticky texture.

2. Then, line an 8x8 baking dish with parchment paper and transfer the crust mixture into the dish. Then, using your

hand, gently press the crust into the bottom of the baking dish and set aside.

3. The next step is to prepare the filling. Add all listed ingredients for the filling to a high-speed blender and blend until the mixture becomes smooth and creamy. Once done, pour the filling mixture on top of the crust and spread evenly.

4. The next step is to prepare the swirl topping. Add all ingredients for the swirl into the food processor and process until the mixture has a puree type texture. Then, drizzle the top of the cake with the filling. Using a sharp knife, swirl the topping into the cheesecake.

5. Then, put the cake in the freezer for at least two hours until it hardens. Once you are ready to serve it, make sure you leave it on the countertop for at least ten minutes, so it softens a bit.

BLUEBERRY ICE CREAM

If you love ice creams, you are going to love this delicious vegan, gluten-free option. This blueberry ice cream will become your favorite icy dessert. This is one of the simplest recipes in the book; so easy to prepare.

Nutritional information for one serving:

- Total Calories: 195
- Protein: 1 grams
- Fat: 10 grams
- Fiber: 0.2 grams
- Carbohydrates: 25 grams

Ingredients:

- 2 cups of frozen blueberries
- 1 avocado
- 1/2 cup of non-dairy yogurt

- 1 teaspoon of vanilla powder
- 1/2 cup of maple syrup or 10 dates
- 1 teaspoon of Maca Powder

Method:

1. Start by adding all listed ingredients to a food processor or blender and pulse until the mixture becomes creamy and thick.

2. Once done, place the blueberry ice cream into a large container and store it in the freezer for one to two hours. Once it is set, scoop it and enjoy.

HEALTHY HOLIDAY FUDGE

If you like simple desserts that come with rich flavors, you will love this wonderfully delectable and healthy holiday fudge that is loaded with rich flavors.

Nutritional information for one serving:

- Total Calories: 115
- Protein: 8 grams
- Fat: 7.2 grams
- Fiber: 3.9 grams
- Carbohydrates: 9 grams

Ingredients:

- 1 cup of organic coconut oil, melted or liquid
- 1/4 cup of organic raw cacao powder
- 1/4 cup of homemade almond butter
- 1/4 cup of organic maple syrup

- 1 tablespoon of vanilla extract

Method:

1. Start with putting all listed ingredients into a medium-sized bowl and stir until all ingredients are well combined.

2. Then, pour the mixture into a 5x9 glass bread pan or into an 8x8 glass baking dish.

3. The next step is to put the pan into the freezer and leave for at least one hour until the mixture is firm. Keep it in the refrigerator until you are ready to serve. Then, cut into fudge squares and enjoy.

PEANUT BUTTER OATMEAL ENERGY BITES

This recipe is very simple requiring only five ingredients to make. Very quickly, you have your peanut butter oatmeal energy bites ready to enjoy. You will love this fast and tasty dessert.

Nutritional information for one serving:

- Total Calories: 120
- Protein: 3 grams
- Fat: 5 grams
- Fiber: 2 grams
- Carbohydrates: 17 grams

Ingredients:

- 1 cup of soft Medjool dates, pitted
- 1 cup of rolled oats, gluten-free

- 1/2 cup of creamy peanut butter, you may use other seeds or nut butter as well
- 1 teaspoon of vanilla extract
- 2-3 tablespoons of water, only if needed to blend

Method:

1. The initial step is to process the Medjool dates in a food processor until the mixture develops a creamy and sticky consistency.

2. Then, add in peanut butter, oats, vanilla and process until all ingredients are well combined.

3. If the dough is dry, add several tablespoons of water to help everything stick together.

4. The next step is to form the dough into small balls using your hands. Once done, place them onto a baking sheet lined with parchment paper. Then, place the pan in the

refrigerator for about thirty minutes to set. Once done, serve and enjoy.

PEANUT BUTTER CHOCOLATE CHIP COOKIES

You will love these flavorful and tasty peanut butter, chocolate chip cookies. After you have tried them, this recipe will become one of your favorites. Prepare a bunch of them as you will want additional servings.

Nutritional information for one serving:

- Total Calories: 310
- Protein: 5 grams
- Fat: 5 grams
- Fiber: 4 grams
- Carbohydrates: 39 grams

Ingredients:

- For dry mix: 1 1/2 cups of brown rice flour
- 2 teaspoons of cornstarch
- 1/2 teaspoon of baking soda
- 2 tablespoons of coconut sugar or cane juice sugar
- For wet mix: 12.68 fl. oz. almond milk or your preferred plant-based milk
- 5 pitted Medjool dates
- 1/2 teaspoon of Celtic sea salt, coarse
- 1 teaspoon of vanilla extract
- 1/4 cup of peanut butter
- For serving: 1/4 cup of vegan chocolate chips

Method:

1. The initial step is to add all dry ingredients to a large mixing bowl. Then, preheat the oven to 375 degrees.

2. The next step is to add all wet ingredients to the blender and pulse until the mixture becomes smooth.

3. Then, add the blended mixture to the dry ingredients mixture and mix thoroughly. Once done, using your hands, mix in the chocolate chips, and combine the entire dough firmly.

4. Using a medium-sized ice cream scoop or spoon, place mixture scoops of cookie dough evenly apart on the baking tray.

5. Put the cookies in the oven for around ten minutes until they become golden brown.

6. Then, let the cookies cool for about five to ten minutes before you serve them.

APPLE CRUMBLE MUFFINS

These tasty apple crumble muffins are loaded with delicious bite-sized pieces of apples. These are high in nutrients, high in fiber, so they are the perfect way to start your day.

Nutritional information for one serving:

- Total Calories: 430
- Protein: 11 grams
- Fat: 13 grams
- Fiber: 9 grams
- Carbohydrates: 60 grams

Ingredients:

- 1 cup of brown rice flour
- 1/2 cup of gluten-free rolled oats
- 1/2 cup of almond meal
- 1/2-3/4 cup of coconut palm sugar

- 2 tablespoons of flax seed meal
- 1 1/2 teaspoons of baking powder
- 1/4 teaspoon of sea salt
- 1 cup of almond milk
- 1 ripe or mashed banana
- 1 teaspoon of vanilla
- 1 apple, peeled and finely diced, you may use extra for garnish
- For garnish: 2 tablespoons of coconut palm sugar
- 2 tablespoons of almond meal
- Pinch of cardamom

Method:

1. The initial step is to preheat the oven to 350 degrees. Then, line a muffin tin with liners.

2. The following step is to mix brown rice flour, almond meal, rolled oats, coconut palm sugar, baking powder, flaxseed meal and sea salt in a large bowl.

3. In a separate bowl, mix the vanilla, banana and almond milk. Then, stir this mixture into the dry mixture and combine well. You may use a wire whisk.

4. The next step is to fold in apple pieces. Once done, spoon the batter evenly into muffin liners.

5. The next step is to combine topping ingredients in a small bowl and sprinkle on top of every muffin. Bake the muffins for about thirty minutes.

6. Once done, transfer the pan to a cooling rack and let muffins cool for five minutes before you serve them. Enjoy.

LAST WORDS

I hope you enjoy preparing and eating these simple, yet tasty vegan, gluten-free recipes that have been illustrated in this book. As you cook them and realize just how satisfying going vegan and gluten-free can make your life, you will notice other changes as well. By following a vegan lifestyle, you will feel more energized, healthier and like nothing can stop you. Losing weight and maintaining a healthy lifestyle is so much more gratifying than just starting a new diet to lose weight.

The other health benefits that you experience from following a vegan, gluten-free diet make going down this path a wonderful and tasty journey almost from the very beginning. In addition, make sure you try the recipes listed here as they can help boost both your mind and body.

Of course, these recipes are not exclusive. They are listed to guide and help on your weight loss journey. As you go through the book and prepare the meals, it's always fun to experiment a bit. Feel free to give those recipes a twist of your own to make them even more appealing to you or your family.

Therefore, grab the book and keep it by your side as you explore appetizing vegan, gluten-free recipes that can be prepared for you and your family in no time. The book will most certainly become your best companion on this adventurous journey. Therefore, keep it near you to consult for the day's menu.

Moreover, and most importantly, do not be afraid of any obstacles that may cross into your path as you take new steps toward your goals as every new step you take brings you closer to a younger, healthier and more energized you.

Printed in Poland
by Amazon Fulfillment
Poland Sp. z o.o., Wrocław